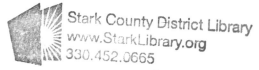

People in My Community

Veterinarians

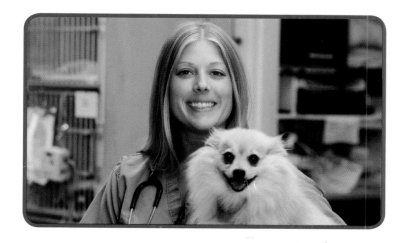

By JoAnn Early Macken

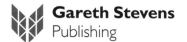

Gareth Stevens
Publishing

Please visit our Web site, www.garethstevens.com. For a free color catalog of all our high-quality books, call toll free 1-800-542-2595 or fax 1-877-542-2596.

Library of Congress Cataloging-in-Publication Data

Macken, JoAnn Early, 1953-
Veterinarians / JoAnn Early Macken.
   p. cm. – (People in my community)
Includes index.
ISBN 978-1-4339-3813-9 (pbk.)
ISBN 978-1-4339-3814-6 (6-pack)
ISBN 978-1-4339-3812-2 (library binding)
1. Veterinarians–Juvenile literature. 2. Veterinary medicine–Juvenile literature. I. Title.
SF756.M232 2011
636.089092–dc22

New edition published 2011 by
Gareth Stevens Publishing
111 East 14th Street, Suite 349
New York, NY 10003

New text and images this edition copyright © 2011 Gareth Stevens Publishing

Original edition published 2003 by Weekly Reader® Books
An imprint of Gareth Stevens Publishing
Original edition text and images copyright © 2003 Gareth Stevens Publishing

Art direction: Haley Harasymiw, Tammy Gruenwald
Page layout: Daniel Hosek, Katherine A. Goedheer
Editorial direction: Kerri O'Donnell, Diane Laska Swanke

Photo credits: Cover, back cover, p. 1 Heidi Schawel/Workbook Stock/Getty Images; pp. 5, 7, 19 © Gregg Andersen; pp. 9, 15, 17, 21 Shutterstock.com; p. 11 Viktor Drachev/AFP/Getty Images; p. 13 Jack Guez/AFP/Getty Images.

Printed in the United States of America

CPSIA compliance information: Batch #CS10GS: For further information contact Gareth Stevens, New York, New York at 1-800-542-2595.

Table of Contents

Meet the Vet! 4

Caring for Pets. 8

Caring for Farm Animals 10

Caring for Wild Animals 12

Special Tools 14

Glossary. 22

For More Information. 23

Index 24

Boldface words appear in the glossary.

Meet the Vet!

A veterinarian is a doctor who takes care of animals. A veterinarian is sometimes called a vet. A vet keeps animals healthy.

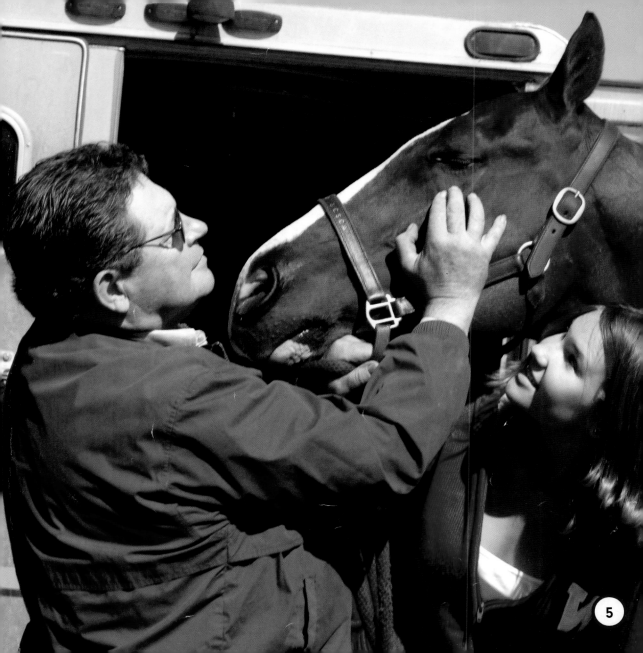

A vet **examines** animals. She gives them **medicine**. She **operates** on them and sets broken bones.

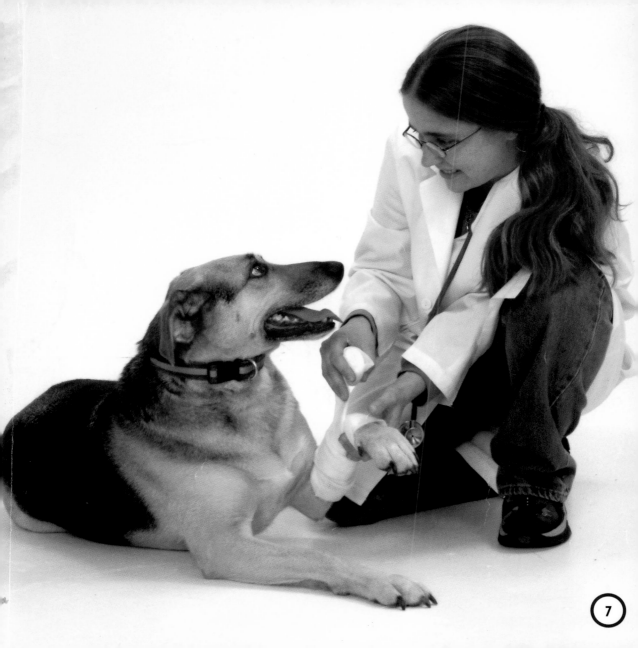

Caring for Pets

Some vets take care of people's pets. Vets may work in an office or an animal **hospital**.

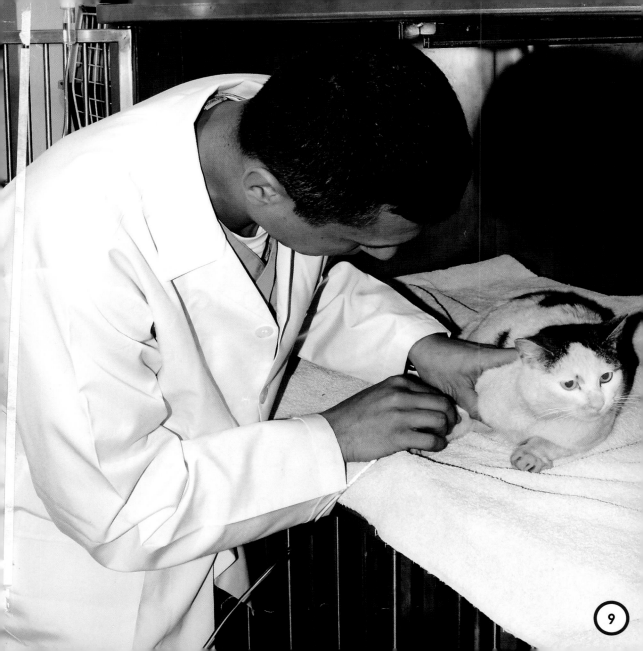

Caring for Farm Animals

Some vets go to farms to treat animals. They help care for horses, cows, sheep, pigs, and other farm animals.

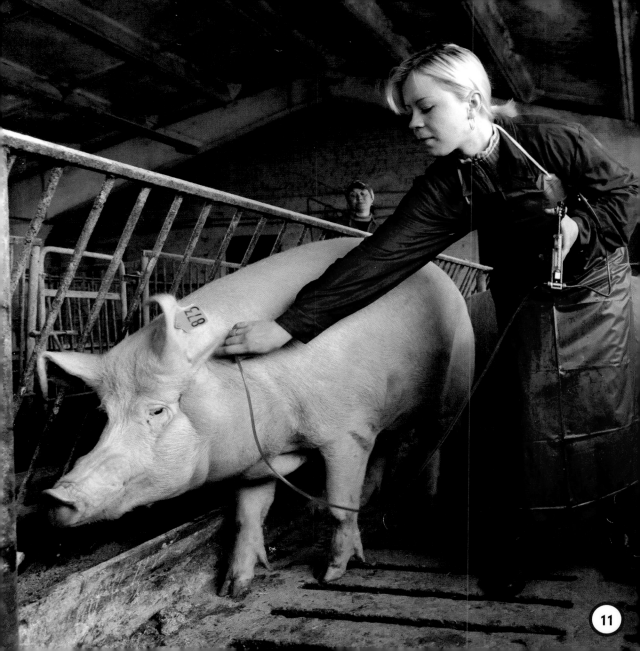

Caring for Wild Animals

Some vets take care of animals that live in the wild. Others take care of wild animals that live at the zoo.

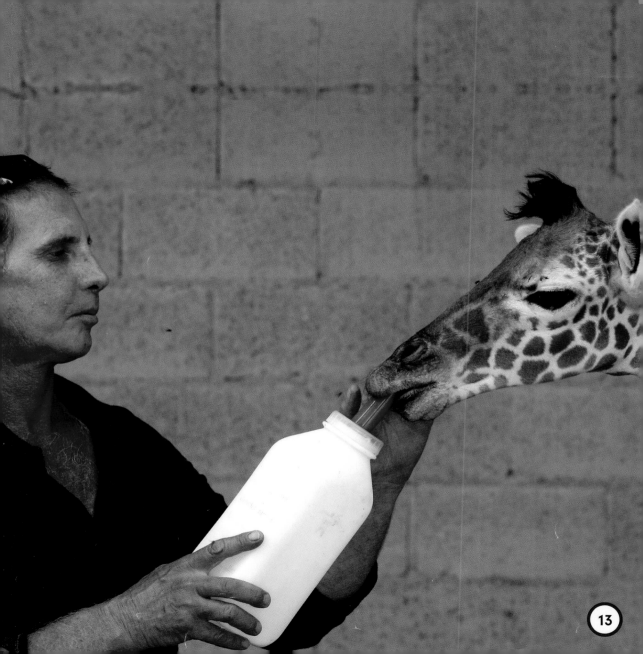

Special Tools

Vets use special tools to care for animals. These tools help them examine an animal's eyes, ears, and mouth.

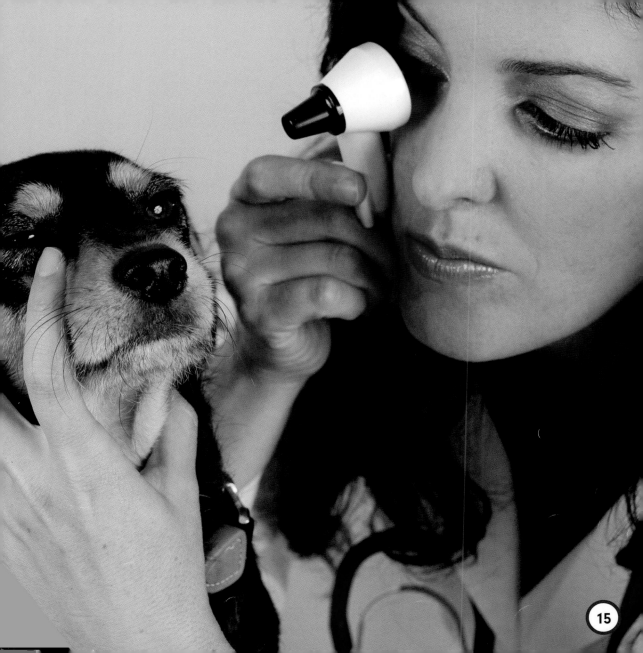

A vet listens to an animal's heartbeat and breathing. To do this, the vet uses a **stethoscope**.

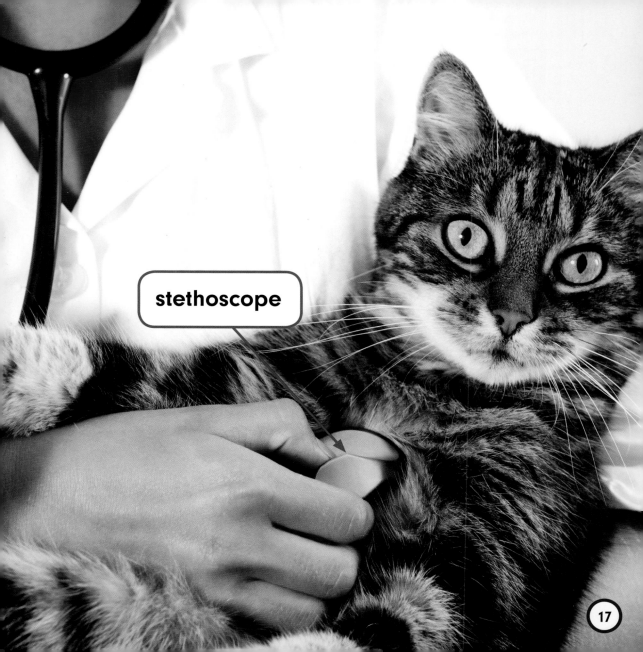

stethoscope

Sometimes a vet needs to take pictures of an animal's bones. He uses a special machine called an **X-ray** machine.

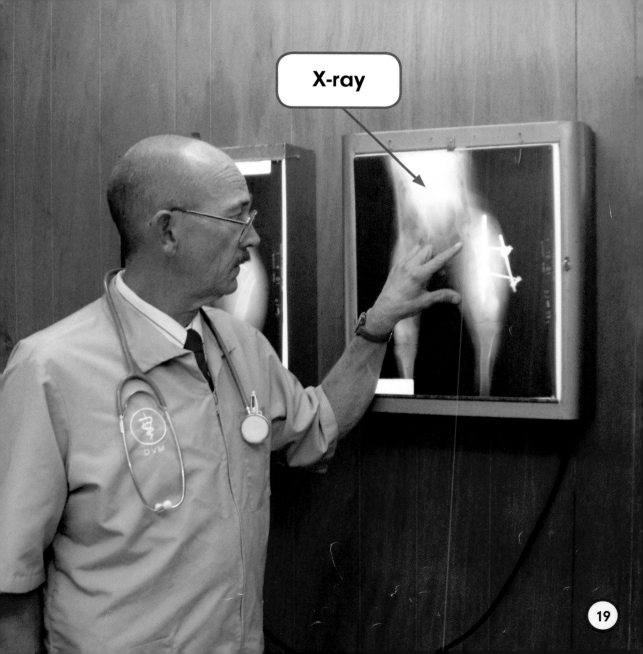

X-ray

Vets show us how to take good care of animals. If you have a question about a pet, ask a vet!

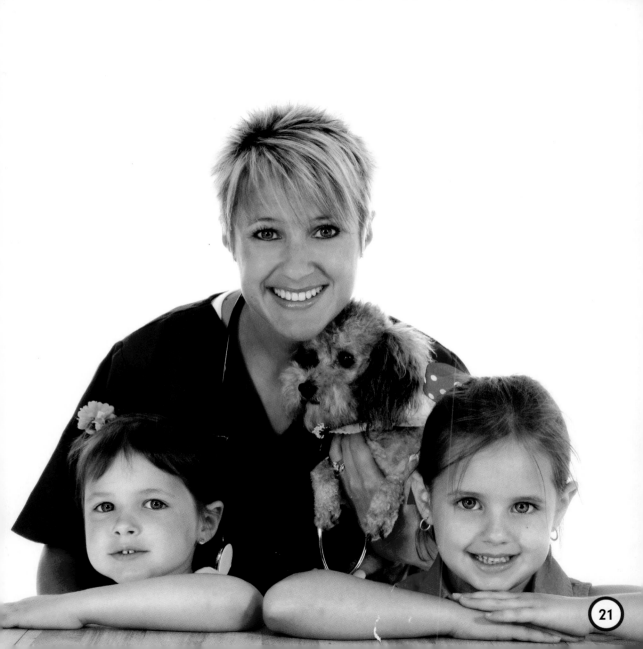

21

Glossary

examine: to look at an animal to see how it is doing

hospital: a place that takes care of sick or hurt animals

medicine: a drug used to fight sickness

operate: to cut open

stethoscope: a tool used to hear the heart and listen to breathing

X-ray: a picture of the inside of something that is taken by a special machine

For More Information

Books

Gregory, Josh. *What Do They Do? Veterinarians*. Ann Arbor, MI: Cherry Lake Publishing, 2010.

Rau, Dana Meachen. *Veterinarian*. New York, NY: Marshall Cavendish Benchmark, 2008.

Web Sites

Care for Animals
www.avma.org/careforanimals/default.asp
Learn about caring for a pet through fun puzzles and games.

FutureVet
www.futurevet.net
Do you want to be a vet? This site shows you what you'll need to do.

Index

animal hospital 8
animals 4, 6, 10, 14, 16, 18, 20
bones 6, 18
cows 10
doctor 4
examines 6, 14
farms 10
healthy 4
horses 10
medicine 6
office 8
operates 6
pets 8, 20
pictures 18
pigs 10
sheep 10
stethoscope 16, 17
tools 14
wild animals 12
X-ray machine 18, 19
zoo 12

About the Author

JoAnn Early Macken is the author of children's poetry; two rhyming picture books, *Cats on Judy* and *Sing-Along Songs*; and various other nonfiction series. She teaches children to write poetry and received the Barbara Juster Esbensen 2000 Poetry Teaching Award. JoAnn is a graduate of the MFA in Writing for Children Program at Vermont College. She lives in Wisconsin with her husband and their two sons.